Autumn Essential Oils:

59 Organic Soaps, Scrubs And Cream Recipes For The Health Of Your Skin + 33 Best Autumn Blends With Essential Oils

Table of content:

Introduction

This book contains amazing recipes to help you make your own homemade natural soap,Scrub, and cream at the convenience of your home! If you're creative at heart, you're definitely a person who likes to dive into new ventures and experiment new things. If this is your first time, worry not! This isn't difficult, the more you practice the more exciting it gets. Once you learn the process of making, you will see how productive, fun and easy it is as a hobby! And once you become a soap, cream, and scrub maker, you will no longer have to worry about buying a product that won't irritate your sensitive skin.

Always wear shoes when you make soap. Never make soap in your bare feet or fancy sandals. Splatters can hurt and irritate your skin, so you want to fully protect yourself. Get a solid pair of shoes that you don't mind getting splattered.

Soap Making Equipment You'll Need

Stainless Steel Pot with a Lid

A 3-12 quart pot allows you to make any size soap you want. While some people may have pots readily available at home (which they can clean thoroughly after the soap-making process and be food ready), others may have to buy one for that purpose.

Handheld Immersion Blender

Much like any handheld blender, immersion blenders are stick-like and have one spinning blade on the end. If you make your own body butters, you know the kind of blender I'm talking about. These blenders will reduce the amount of stirring time, making your life easier!

Spoon or Whisk and Spatula

Stay away from wooden spoons: use stainless steel instead! I tried using my favorite wooden spoon and over time little wood splinters ended up in my soap bar. As with the spatula, my mantra is stainless steel is the best.

Bowls

For weighing oils, butters, water, or lye, I use stainless steel and plastic bowls with lids. I once had to clean up a lot of mess after one of my bowls tipped over, pouring everything on my shoes! From then on, I decided to use bowls I could close with lids to avoid extra work!

Plastic Pitcher with a Lid

I use a plastic pitcher to mix lye. One time I used a glass pitcher and the mixture etched the glass (it **nearly exploded!**), and I had to say goodbye to what could have been a lovely masterpiece on my dining table! Remember that lye heats up, so use something that will bear the heat.

Scale

If you're just starting out, you need a scale to measure the right amount of ingredients. I bought a kitchen scale with a flat platform so I can place my bowls and pitchers on it to see if I'm right on track with the measurements. Buy a scale that also measures in grams – it is important, trust me.

Stainless Steel Thermometer

With a thermometer, you'll be able to tell the temperature of the oils and lye or water so you'll know when to mix certain ingredients. The oils need to be very hot for the soap to set up; and because you can't put your finger in to check the heat, you need a thermometer!

Soap Molds

You'll need a non-aluminum, preferably plastic container that will produce the shape of your soap. Once you're done making your soap mixture, you can pour it into your soap molds to create rectangular, square, circle, or any shape of soap you like.

Other Optional Stuff

You need old towels to keep the soap warm when poured into the molds, and a vegetable cutter to cut out the uneven sides of your soap.

What about the Shelf Life?

This really depends on the additives you add to your soap. Some of my soaps are five years old! If you add essential oils, the shelf life will be reduced because they often don't stay well in soap. What you should know is that the shelf life of any soap depends particularly on the iodine value. For example, if the soap has too much iodine, some orange spots will appear on the soap – an indication that it is going bad. If you use the right amount of iodine, your soap will remain good for a long, long time.

Chapter 1. Organic Soap Recipes

Dish soap

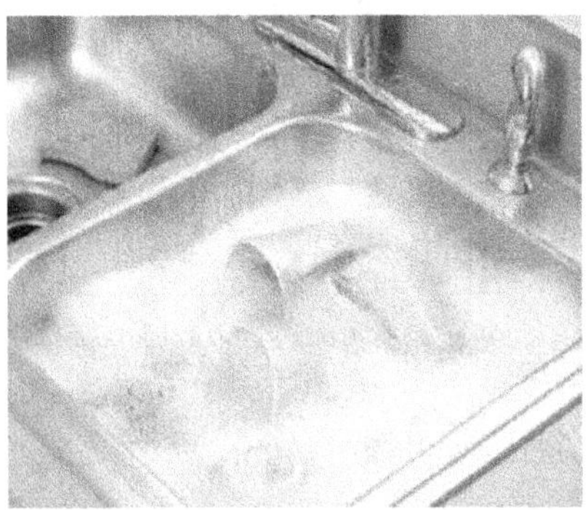

12 Ounces Coconut oil 76 Degree

21.6 Ounces Olive oil

14.4 Ounces Palm oil

.75 ounces Lemon Essential oil

.75 ounces of Tea Tree oil

7.10 ounces Lye (sodium hydroxide)

15.84 water

Large Crock Pot

• Place the measured oils in the crock pot.

• Slowly add the lye to the water and stir carefully until it dissolves. The solution will get hot. Be sure to insulate your hands.

• While you are mixing the oils with the mixer, slowly pour the lye solution into the crock pot. It's best to do this away from you have the mixer.

• Mix all the ingredients with the mixer until you see it leave trails in the compound. This is tracing.

- Cover the crock pot and set a timer for 25 minutes.
- After 25 minutes, lift the lid and stir again, this time adding the essential oils.
- Test with a litmus strip. Cover set timer another ten minutes.
- Test again if the compound came back acidic. Stir with a spatula. If it pulls away from the side of the crock pot, it is ready to be put in a mold to finish curing.
- Allow to sit overnight.

To Use

Grate 4 ounce of soap at a time through a blender and process until fine. Add a 1/4 cup to running water before you wash your dishes. Just agitate the water if you see the suds disappearing. Because there are no phosphates in the soap to prolong the suds, the bubbles will dissipate faster.

All Purpose Clothes Detergent

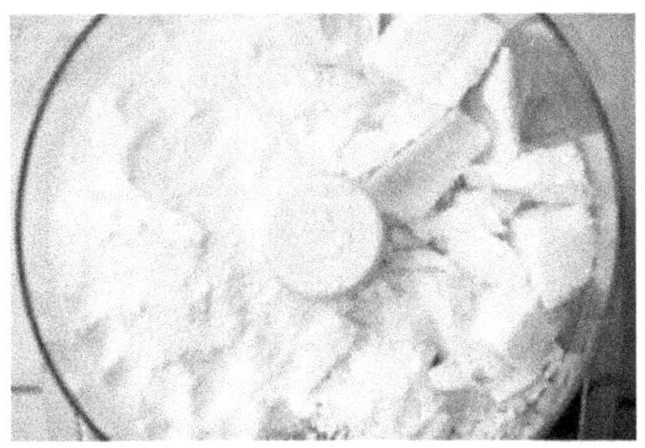

12 ounces of Coconut oil 76 degree

14.4 ounces Palm oil

7.2 Ounces of Palm Kernel Flakes

14.4 Ounces of Olive Oil

.75 Ounces Orange Blossom Essential oil

.75 Ounces of Tea Tree Essential oil

7.42 ounces lye (sodium hydroxide)

15.84 ounces water

1 cup baking soda

1 cup Borax

1 cup hydrogen booster

Large Crock Pot

- Mix the last three ingredients together and set them aside.
- Make the soap as listed above.
- Finely grate 4 ounces of the soap into a food processor and add the other ingredients.
- Place the detergent in a tightly lidded container when not in use.
- Use 1 tablespoon per regular load, 2 if it's a particularly dirty load.

Baby detergent

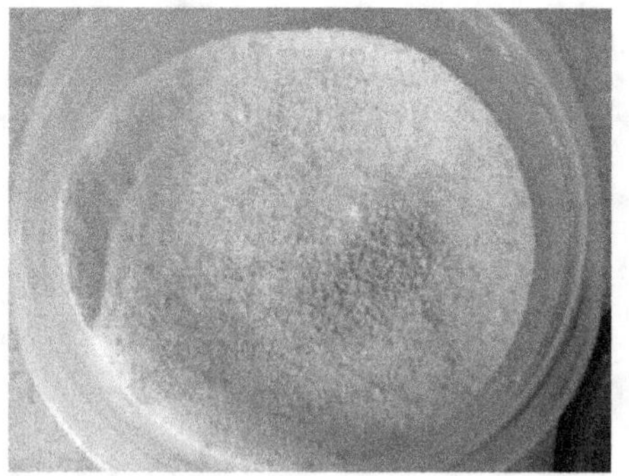

12 ounces of Coconut oil 76 degree

14.4 ounces Palm oil

21.6 Ounces of Olive Oil

7.10 Ounces Lye

15.84 Ounces water

1.5 Ounces Lavender Essential

1 cup baking soda

1 cup Borax

Large Crock Pot

Follow the same instructions as above.

Floor Cleaner

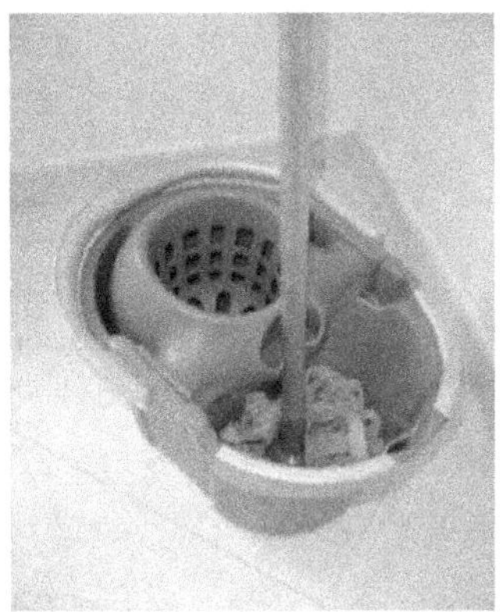

12 ounces of Coconut oil 76 degree

14.4 ounces Palm oil

7.2 Ounces of Palm Kernel Flakes

14.4 Ounces of Olive Oil

7.42 ounces lye

15.84 ounces water

.75 Tea Tree Essential Oil

.75 Lemon Essential Oil

1 cup baking soda

1 cup Borax

1 cup hydrogen booster

Large Crock Pot

Follow directions as the clothing detergent, but use 1/4 cup of the cleaner in three gallons of hot water.

Soaps for Him

Chemistry is important when making soaps. A man's chemistry is vastly different from a woman's and that is what are addressing in this chapter with these essential oils and soap recipes.

Essential Oils

From the list in the last chapter, we have *Tea Tree* and *Lemon*. Here is a list of others that are also good for deodorant purposes are:

Thyme: This is a woody herb that can help curve body odor.

Rosemary: This is another herbal essential oil that mixes well with a man's chemistry. Not to be used if you suffer from hypertension.

Sandalwood: This is a musky essential oil that mixes with a man's chemistry.

Cypress: This is an essential oil that is really good for controlling perspiration.

Body odor I

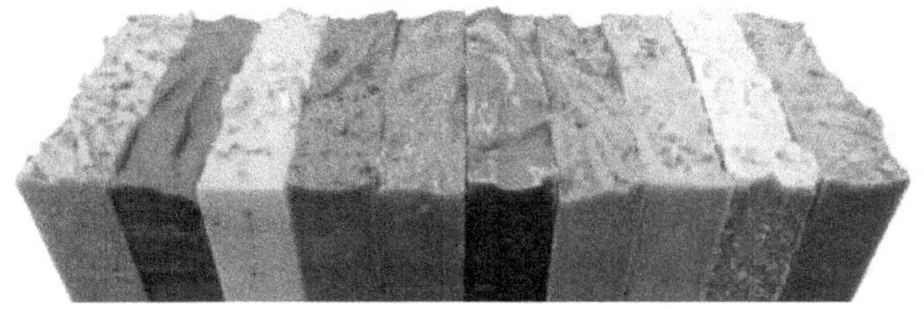

12 Ounces of Coconut Oil

36 Ounces Olive Oil

6.96 ounces lye

15.84 Water

.50 oz Tea Tree Essential Oil

.50 oz Cypress Essential Oil

.50 oz Thyme Essential Oil

Body Odor II

12 Ounces of Coconut Oil

36 Ounces Olive Oil

6.96 ounces lye

15.84 Water

.50 oz Sandalwood Essential Oil

.50 oz Lemon Essential Oil

.50 oz Rosemary Essential Oil

Mechanics Soap

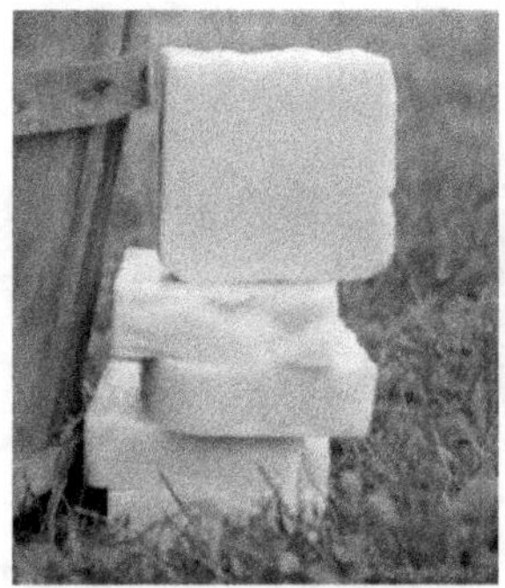

I know this sounds likes a silly name for a soap, but if you work a dirty or oily job, you need a soap that will do the trick.

12 Ounces Coconut Oil 76 Degrees

14.4 Ounces of Palm Oil

21.6 Ounces Olive Oil

7.84 Ounces lye

15.84 Ounces water

.50 oz Tea Tree Essential Oil

.50 oz Cypress Essential Oil

.50 oz Lemon Essential Oil

1/2 Cup Pumice Powder

1/4 Cup Kelp Powder (Skin conditioner)

Follow the directions on making the soap

Mechanics Soap II

12 Ounces Coconut Oil 76 Degrees

14.4 Ounces of Palm Oil

21.6 Ounces Olive Oil

7.84 Ounces lye

15.84 Ounces water

.50 oz Sandalwood Essential Oil

.50 oz Cypress Essential Oil

.50 oz Orange Blossom Essential Oil

3/4 Cup Pumice Powder

Facial Cleansing

12 Ounces Coconut Oil 76 Degrees

4.8 Ounces Jojoba Oil

7.2 Ounces Palm Kernel Flakes

14.4 Palm oil

9.6 Ounces of Olive Oil

7.11 Ounces lye

15.84 Ounces water

.75 oz Lemon Essential Oil (for cutting oils)

.75 oz Myrrh Essential Oil (cracked skin)

Facial Scrubber

This is a cleanser for men that has an exfoliant in it.

12 Ounces Coconut Oil 76 Degrees

4.8 Ounces Jojoba Oil

7.2 Ounces Palm Kernel Flakes

14.4 Palm oil

9.6 Ounces of Olive Oil

7.11 Ounces lye

15.84 Ounces water

1/2 Cup Kelp powder

.50 oz Sandalwood Essential Oil

.50 oz Lemon Essential Oil

.50 oz Tea Tree Oil

Dry Scalp Shampoo

12 Ounces Coconut Oil 76 Degrees

4.8 Ounces Jojoba Oil

7.2 Ounces Palm Kernel Flakes

14.4 Palm oil

9.6 Ounces of Olive Oil

7.11 Ounces lye

15.84 Ounces water

.50 oz Sandalwood Essential Oil

.50 oz Lavender Essential Oil

.50 oz Myrrh Essential Oil (Helps moisturize scalp)

1/4 cup Olive Oil

Filtered Water

When the soap is done curing:

- Grate the soap into a blender
- Add the oil
- Set the blender to blend and add water until it reaches a shampoo consistency.

Oily Hair Shampoo

12 Ounces Coconut Oil 76 Degrees

4.8 Ounces Jojoba Oil

7.2 Ounces Palm Kernel Flakes

14.4 Palm oil

9.6 Ounces of Olive Oil

7.11 Ounces lye

15.84 Ounces water

.50 oz Lemon Essential Oil

.50 oz Orange Blossom Essential Oil

.50 oz Cypress Essential Oil

Soaps for Her

In this chapter, we will go over all the soap products that a woman can use.

Body odor

12 Ounces of Coconut Oil

36 Ounces Olive Oil

6.96 ounces lye

15.84 Water

.50 oz Lavender Essential Oil

.50 oz Cypress Essential Oil

.50 oz Peppermint Essential Oil

Soothing Soap

12 Ounces of Coconut Oil

36 Ounces Olive Oil

6.96 ounces lye

15.84 Water

.50 oz Lavender Essential Oil

.50 oz Rosewood (Soothes the nerves and skin)

.50 oz Orange Blossom Essential Oil

Exfoliating Soap

12 Ounces of Coconut Oil

36 Ounces Olive Oil

6.96 ounces lye

15.84 Water

3/4 Cup Kelp Powder

.50 oz Lemon Essential oil

.50 oz Rosewood Essential Oil

.50 oz Roman Chamomile Essential Oil

Scrubbing Soap

12 Ounces of Coconut Oil

36 Ounces Olive Oil

6.96 ounces lye

15.84 Water

3/4 Cup Sea Salt

.50 oz Peppermint Essential Oil

.50 oz Lemon Essential Oil

.50 oz Geranium Essential Oil

Dry Skin I

12 Ounces Coconut Oil 76 Degrees

9.6 Ounces Hemp Seed Oil

4.8 Ounces Jojoba Oil

7.2 Ounces Palm Kernel Oil

14.4 Ounces Olive Oil

6.44 Ounces lye

14.85 Ounces water

.50 oz Palmarosa Essential Oil (Great for softening skin)

.50 oz Lavender Essential Oil

.50 oz Orange Blossom Essential Oil

Dry Skin II Mature Skin

12 Ounces Coconut Oil 76 Degrees

9.6 Ounces Hemp Seed Oil

4.8 Ounces Jojoba Oil

7.2 Ounces Palm Kernel Oil

14.4 Ounces Olive Oil

6.44 Ounces lye

14.85 Ounces water

.50 oz Myrrh Essential Oil

.50 oz Orange Blossom Essential Oil

.50 oz Rose Essential Oil (Tones mature skin)

Shampoo I (oily hair)

7.2 Ounces Apricot Kernel Oil

12 Ounces Coconut Oil 76 Degrees

9.6 Ounces Hemp Seed Oil

4.8 Ounces Jojoba Oil

14.4 Ounces Olive Oil

6.66 Ounces lye

15.84 Ounces of water

.50 oz Orange Blossom Essential Oil

.50 oz Grapefruit Essential Oil

.50 oz Lavender Essential Oil

1/4 Cup Sweet Almond oil

Filtered

- Make the soap as normal.
- Grate 4 ounces of the soap into a blender
- Add the Almond oil and put it on the blend setting.
- Add water to the mixture until it is a shampoo consistency.
- You may have to shake the shampoo to mix it. It will separate.

Soaps for Kids

Home made lye soaps are not recommended for infants to toddlers. To be on the safe side, it is alright to use these types of soaps on children 5 years and older.

Boys can get really dirty. Sometimes it seems you can bathe them, dress them in nice clothes, sneeze, and they're dirty all over again. Here are a couple of recipes that can help clean them up.

Boys' Soap I

12 Ounces Coconut oil 76 Degrees

26.40 Ounces Olive Oil

9.6 Ounces Palm Oil

7.06 Ounces lye

15.84 Ounces water

.50 oz Cedarwood Essential Oil (for the skin)

.50 oz Cypress Essential Oil (perspiration and body odor)

.50 oz Orange Blossom Essential Oil

Boys' Soap II

12 Ounces Coconut oil 76 Degrees

9.6 Ounces Hemp Seed Oil

2.4 Ounces Olive Oil

14.4 Ounces Palm Oil

9.6 Ounces Olive Oil

7.13 Ounces lye

15.84 Ounces of water

.50 oz Rosewood Essential Oil (sensitive skin, young skin)

.50 oz Chamomile Essential Oil

.50 oz Mandarin Essential Oil

Girls' Soap I

12 Ounces Coconut Oil 76 Degrees

7.2 Ounces Grapeseed Oil

9.6 Ounces Hemp Seed Oil

4.8 Ounces Olive Oil

14.4 Ounces Palm Oil

7.11 Ounces lye

15.84 Ounces water

.50 oz Lavender Essential Oil

.50 oz Orange Blossom Essential Oil

.50 oz Roman Chamomile Essential Oil

Girls' Soap II

12 Ounces Coconut Oil 76 Degrees

7.2 Ounces Grapeseed Oil

9.6 Ounces Hemp Seed Oil

4.8 Ounces Olive Oil

14.4 Ounces Palm Oil

7.11 Ounces lye

15.84 Ounces water

.50 oz Geranium Essential Oil

.50 oz Cypress Essential Oil

.50 oz Rosewood Essential Oil

Boys' Facial Cleanser I (oily skin)

12 Ounces Coconut oil 76 Degrees

26.40 Ounces Olive Oil

9.6 Ounces Palm Oil

7.06 Ounces lye

15.84 Ounces water

.75 oz Frankincense Essential Oil

.75 oz Mandarin Essential Oil (for oily skin)

Boys' Facial Cleanser II (dry skin)

12 Ounces Coconut Oil 76 Degrees

7.2 Ounces Grapeseed Oil

9.6 Ounces Hemp Seed Oil

4.8 Ounces Olive Oil

14.4 Ounces Palm Oil

7.11 Ounces lye

15.84 Ounces water

.50 oz Lavender Essential oil (blemishes)

.50 oz Rosewood Essential Oil

.50 oz Cypress Essential Oil

Girls' Facial Cleanser (oily skin)

12 Ounces Coconut Oil 76 Degrees

7.2 Ounces Grapeseed Oil

9.6 Ounces Hemp Seed Oil

4.8 Ounces Olive Oil

14.4 Ounces Palm Oil

7.11 Ounces lye

15.84 Ounces water

.75 oz Lavender Essential Oil

.75 oz Orange Blossom Essential Oil

Girls' Facial Cleanser II (Dry Skin)

12 Ounces Coconut Oil 76 Degrees

7.2 Ounces Grapeseed Oil

9.6 Ounces Hemp Seed Oil

4.8 Ounces Olive Oil

14.4 Ounces Palm Oil

7.11 Ounces lye

15.84 Ounces water

.75 oz Rose Otto Essential Oil

.75 oz Rosewood Essential Oil

Other Soaps

Soothing Soap

12 Ounces of Coconut Oil

36 Ounces Olive Oil

6.96 ounces lye

15.84 Water

.50 oz Lavender Essential Oil

.50 oz Rosewood (Soothes the nerves and skin)

.50 oz Orange Blossom Essential Oil

Exfoliating Soap

12 Ounces of Coconut Oil

36 Ounces Olive Oil

6.96 ounces lye

15.84 Water

3/4 Cup Kelp Powder

.50 oz Lemon Essential oil

.50 oz Rosewood Essential Oil

.50 oz Roman Chamomile Essential Oil

Scrubbing Soap

12 Ounces of Coconut Oil

36 Ounces Olive Oil

6.96 ounces lye

15.84 Water

3/4 Cup Sea Salt

.50 oz Peppermint Essential Oil

.50 oz Lemon Essential Oil

.50 oz Geranium Essential Oil

Dry Skin I

12 Ounces Coconut Oil 76 Degrees

9.6 Ounces Hemp Seed Oil

4.8 Ounces Jojoba Oil

7.2 Ounces Palm Kernel Oil

14.4 Ounces Olive Oil

6.44 Ounces lye

14.85 Ounces water

.50 oz Palmarosa Essential Oil (Great for softening skin)

.50 oz Lavender Essential Oil

.50 oz Orange Blossom Essential Oil

Dry Skin II Mature Skin

12 Ounces Coconut Oil 76 Degrees

9.6 Ounces Hemp Seed Oil

4.8 Ounces Jojoba Oil

7.2 Ounces Palm Kernel Oil

14.4 Ounces Olive Oil

6.44 Ounces lye

14.85 Ounces water

.50 oz Myrrh Essential Oil

.50 oz Orange Blossom Essential Oil

.50 oz Rose Essential Oil (Tones mature skin)

Shampoo I (oily hair)

7.2 Ounces Apricot Kernel Oil

12 Ounces Coconut Oil 76 Degrees

9.6 Ounces Hemp Seed Oil

4.8 Ounces Jojoba Oil

14.4 Ounces Olive Oil

6.66 Ounces lye

15.84 Ounces of water

.50 oz Orange Blossom Essential Oil

.50 oz Grapefruit Essential Oil

.50 oz Lavender Essential Oil

1/4 Cup Sweet Almond oil

Filtered

- Make the soap as normal.
- Grate 4 ounces of the soap into a blender
- Add the Almond oil and put it on the blend setting.
- Add water to the mixture until it is a shampoo consistency.
- You may have to shake the shampoo to mix it. It will separate.

Dry/Frizzy Hair

7.2 Ounces Apricot Kernel Oil

12 Ounces Coconut Oil 76 Degrees

9.6 Ounces Hemp Seed Oil

4.8 Ounces Jojoba Oil

14.4 Ounces Olive Oil

6.66 Ounces lye

15.84 Ounces of water

.50 oz Rosewood Essential oil

.50 oz Rosemary Essential oil

.50 oz Palmarosa Essential oil

(All three are wonderful for conditioning the hair and scalp.)

1/4 Argon oil

Filtered Water

Follow the instructions for thc shampoo above.

Facial Cleanser (Dry Skin)

12 Ounces Coconut oil 76 Degrees

9.6 Ounces Hemp Seed Oil

2.4 Ounces Olive Oil

14.4 Ounces Palm Oil

9.6 Ounces Olive Oil

7.13 Ounces lye

15.84 Ounces of water

.50 oz Lavender Essential Oil

.50 oz Chamomile Essential Oil

.50 oz Rosewood Essential Oil

Oily Skin Cleanser

12 Ounces Coconut oil 76 Degrees

9.6 Ounces Hemp Seed Oil

2.4 Ounces Olive Oil

14.4 Ounces Palm Oil

9.6 Ounces Olive Oil

7.13 Ounces lye

15.84 Ounces of water

.50 oz Orange Blossom Essential oil

.50 oz Neroli Essential Oil (for skin toning and balance)

.50 oz Galbanum (balances the skin)

Chapter 2. Scrub Recipes

You have seen many scrubs in the store for your body and face. You have seen the results of using them, but the problem you would like to save money by making your own. You've looked all over the internet to find information on how to make scrubs on your own, but the flood of information is difficult to parse and find just what you are looking for in order to get started.

Scrubs can smooth rough spots on elbows and knees. They can also help to lightly scrub off dead skin from the face and other areas well. It can also moisturize your skin as well.

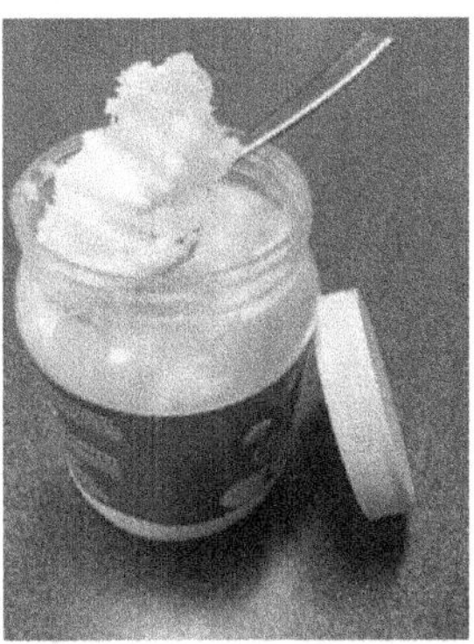

What you need...

There are a few simple things you will need to get started on your new hobby.

□ Glass mixing bowls: You will need two of these to keep the dry ingredients separate from the wet ones until you are ready to mix them.

□ Measuring cups: This is for measuring the sugar and other ingredients you will need.

□ Wooden or glass spoons for mixing

□ Airtight containers to store your scrubs

□ Oils to mix into your scrubs

□ Sugar, white or brown, preferably organic

□ Essential oils

□ Gloves to protect your hands while mixing

No doubt many of you have seen me type both "greasy" and "oily skin". There is a slight difference between the two. Oily skin tends to maintain a sheen on your face which is steady throughout the day, making you constantly check your makeup to cover those "shiny spots". Greasy skin is a more severe form of oily skin. Greasy skin produces more oils, making it impossible to go through a day and not have to wash your face to get rid of the excess oils.

There are ways of combatting oily/greasy skin besides washing your face and using scrubs:

1. Moisturize your skin. I know this may seem like you are adding oils to an already oily situation, but a nice and light moisturizer can prevent your skin from pulling in or producing too much oil to keep itself from drying out.

2. Keep a food diary. Even though many may say what you eat will not affect your skin, not all body chemistry is the same. One person can eat as much chocolate as they want and never have a skin problem while another, figuratively, breaks out just by looking at the confection.

3. Don't overdo it with washing your face. Keeping you face clean is a good idea, but if you are washing your face more than twice a day, you may be washing it too much. Your skin needs to produce some natural oils to maintain a pH balance, and when you are constantly washing your skin, you're forcing it to over compensate.

Chocolate Scrub

Cocoa not only smells divine, but it is also fantastic for the skin. Chocolate masks and baths have become popular due to cocoa's inherent antioxidant capabilities. When applied to the skin, these help to rid the body of skin-damaging free radicals.

Makes: 16 ounces

Ingredients

3 tablespoons organic cocoa powder

1 teaspoon cocoa essential oil

1 ¼ cups organic cane sugar

¾ cup coconut oil

Directions

1.   Combine the ingredients in an airtight jar, mix well, and store in a cool place.

2.   Moisten the skin and scrub with the mixture, wash off.

Coffee Scrub

Now you can have your coffee and drink it too, with this wonderfully aromatic coffee scrub made out of coffee grounds! The coffee grounds stimulate the skin. It's also believed that rubbing the grounds on cellulite helps to reduce it!

Makes: 12 ounces

Ingredients

½ cup coffee grounds
1 cup coconut oil
1 teaspoon vanilla extract

Directions

1.   Combine the ingredients in an airtight jar, mix well, and store in a cool place.

2.   Moisten the skin and scrub with the mixture, wash off.

Lemon Scrub

Drop a little lemon into your scrub, and you'll see it do amazing things for your skin – like magic. Rub the lemony scrub onto your elbows and knees and watch the dark spots disappear! Additionally, lemon's astringent properties help to truly clean the skin and make it brighter.

Makes: 12 ounces

Ingredients

2 teaspoons lemon peel, grated
1 tablespoon lemon juice
1 cup organic cane sugar
2 teaspoons vitamin E oil
½ cup coconut oil

Directions

1.　Combine the ingredients in an airtight jar, mix well, and store in a cool place.

2.　Moisten the skin and scrub with the mixture, wash off.

Mint Chocolate Scrub

Scrub this on your body in the morning, and be prepared to have the wheels in your head turning at ultimate speeds all day! The scent of peppermint has a big, positive affect on mental function in ways such as improving memory and focus.

Makes: 12 ounces

Ingredients

1 cup organic cane sugar
½ cup almond oil
2 tablespoons pure cocoa powder
1 teaspoon peppermint essential oil

Directions

1.   Combine the ingredients in an airtight jar, mix well, and store in a cool place.

2.   Moisten the skin and scrub with the mixture, wash off.

Epsom Foot Scrub

Dry, hardened spots on the skin are terrible to touch and pretty horrible to look at. They can be disheartening personally and quite embarrassing. This is why you must absolutely use this scrub to make your feet beautiful and lovely. Epsom salt is anti-fungal and helps to deodorize feet. In addition, the minerals also help to alleviate pain and discomfort. Your feet work hard for you, so it is definitely time to show them some love.

Makes: 12 ounces

Ingredients

¾ cup Epsom salt
¼ cup sea salt
½ cup coconut oil

Directions

1.   Combine the ingredients in an airtight jar, mix well, and store in a cool place.

2.   Moisten the skin and scrub with the mixture, wash off.

Rice and Honey Whitening Body Scrub

Rice powder has excellent exfoliating properties, and it also helps in brightening skin tone. Honey is one of the best organic applications for your skin. It works as an antibacterial and anti-aging product. It opens up the pores and it is a good natural moisturizer that soothes your skin. It makes your skin glow, and makes it soft and supple to touch.

Makes: 12 ounces

Ingredients

1 cup rice, coarsely ground
3 tablespoons honey
10-12 drops almond oil (use only for dry skin)

Directions

1.   Combine the ingredients in an airtight jar, mix well, and store in a cool place.

2.   Moisten the skin and scrub with the mixture for a couple of minutes, then wash it off.

Summer Red Lentil Body Scrub

Rose water helps you feel refreshed during summertime. It provides relief for itchiness or a burning sensation. Honey is a good moisturizer, an antioxidant, and an antibacterial too. It suits all types of skin and makes your skin supple. The red lentils help remove dead skin cells from your skin and also give to add a healthy glow.

Makes: 12 ounces

Ingredients

½ cup red lentils, coarsely ground
3 tablespoons honey
2 tablespoons rose water

Directions

1.   Combine ingredients in an airtight jar, mix well and store in a cool place.

2.   Moisten skin and scrub with mixture, wash off.

Red Lentil Body Scrub for Winter

Winter can rob your skin of its natural moisture. If you have dry skin, then moisturizing frequently is important. That is where organic ghee comes to the rescue – a heavy duty natural skin moisturizer. It works wonders on dry skin, making it soft and supple. The red lentils help remove dead skin cells and also give you a healthy glow.

Makes: 12 ounces

Ingredients

1 cup red lentils, coarsely ground
½ cup ghee
Rose essential oil (since ghee can have a strong aroma)

Directions

1.   Combine the ingredients in an airtight jar, mix well, and store in a cool place.

2.   Moisten the skin and scrub with the mixture, wash off.

Glowing Soft Skin Body Scrub

This body scrub is full of goodness. Aloe Vera works wonders for moisturizing your skin, and it works very well on dry skin in particular. It is a good skin conditioner and is rich in vitamin E. It also nourishes your skin and helps prevent wrinkles. Walnuts are loaded with vitamins and minerals that are great for the skin, and almonds are good source of vitamin E, which prevents wrinkles and gives a healthy glow to your skin. Honey is a great moisturizer for all types of skin.

Makes: 6 ounces Preparation time: 5 minutes

Ingredients

1 leaf of aloe vera
2 walnuts, in the shell
2 almonds, in the shell
2 tablespoons honey

Directions

1.   Remove the pulp from the aloe vera leaf.

2.   Grind all the ingredients together to get a coarse paste.

3.   Apply the mixture to the skin, and leave it on for 5 minutes. Scrub lightly in circular motions.

4.   Wash it off with lukewarm water.

5.   Always make the scrub fresh and use. Discard leftovers. Use it once a week for soft and supple skin.

Face Whitening Scrub for Dry Skin

Milk is a natural skin moisturizer, and it's great for dry skin. People with oily skin should avoid this scrub, as it will make your face oilier. Rice powder helps in getting rid of dead skin cells and is also known to whiten your skin tone. This scrub is best used at night.

Makes: 12 ounces

Ingredients

½ cup rice, coarsely powdered
½ cup lukewarm milk

Directions

1.   Mix the rice powder and milk together in a bowl to form a paste.

2.   Before bed, apply it on the face and scrub in a circular motion.

3.   Wash it off with lukewarm water. Your face may feel a bit oily for the time being, but the natural oils from the milk will be absorbed into your skin, and you will be left with a fresh and dewy face the next morning.

Lemon Lavender Body Scrub

Scrubs are not just for getting rid of dead skin cells. Body scrubs are also known to help relieve tension and help the body relax. Epsom salt, when used in a scrub, relaxes your muscles and also helps reduce inflammation. Olive oil keeps the skin moist. Lemon juice acts as a bleaching agent, while the lavender helps you relax your senses. Used all together, this relaxing body scrub is just what you need for both body and mind after a tough day.

Makes: 12 ounces

Ingredients

1 ¼ cups Epsom salt or coarse salt crystals
¼ cup olive oil
¼ cup lemon juice
10 drops lavender essential oil

Directions

1.   Combine the ingredients in an airtight jar, mix well, and store in a cool place.

2.   Moisten the skin and scrub with the mixture, wash off.

Anti-inflammatory Body Scrub

Turmeric has anti-inflammatory and antibacterial properties that soothe your skin and help fight skin bacteria. Essential oils (depending on the type you choose) have their own skincare and relaxation benefits. Sugar and salt will help get rid of dead skin cells.

Makes: 25 ounces

Ingredients

1 ½ cups salt
1 ½ cups sugar
3 tablespoons turmeric powder
6-8 drops essential oil of your choice

Directions

1.   Combine the ingredients in an airtight jar, mix well, and store in a cool place.

2.   Moisten the skin and scrub with the mixture, wash off.

Scrub for Sensitive Skin

Avocado is rich in natural oils that help moisturize skin. Cucumber is known for its oil removal properties and is also a natural coolant. It has skin whitening properties as well, and it gives relief to burns and other skin inflammations. Brown sugar is an excellent dead skin cell remover.

Makes: 12 ounces

Ingredients

1 medium cucumber, chopped
1 cup brown sugar
½ cup avocado oil

Directions

1.	Blend the cucumber pieces in a blender until smooth.

2.	In a bowl, combine the blended cucumber, avocado oil, and brown sugar.

3.	Rub the mixture gently all over your body. Leave it on for 3-4 minutes.

4.	Wash with lukewarm water.

Scrub for Soothing Sore Muscles

Epsom salt is known to soothe sore muscles because it contains magnesium. This invigorating combination of Epsom salt with shea butter and essential oils is sure to help remove stiffness and tension from your hard-working body.

Makes: 12 ounces

Ingredients

⅓ cup raw shea butter

¼ cup olive oil

½ teaspoon tangerine essential oil

20 drops lavender essential oil

20 drops eucalyptus essential oil

1 cup Epsom salts

Directions

1. Place the shea butter in a heatproof bowl and melt it in the microwave at 50% power.

2. Add the olive oil and mix.

3. Add the essential oils one at a time, mixing after each addition.

4. Pour in the Epsom salts and mix thoroughly.

5. To use, massage the scrub over sore muscles and rinse off. A scoop may be added to bathwater for a soothing soak.

Apple Spice Scrub

Gently exfoliate while leaving your skin smooth and soft, with the comforting scent of apple and cinnamon.

Makes: 20 ounces

Ingredients

1 cup of sugar
1 cup brown sugar
1 teaspoon apple pie spice
1 teaspoon cinnamon
½ - ¾ cup of coconut oil
6-10 drops apple essential oil (optional)

Directions

1.   Combine all the ingredients together and mix well.

2.   Massage on the skin and rinse off.

__Anti-Cellulite Scrub__

Take your basic coffee scrub to a higher level by adding sugar for better stimulation. This improves circulation, and with coffee's anti-cellulite and tightening effects, you'll have softer, smoother, younger-looking skin. The vanilla has anti-inflammatory properties, while its aroma helps you to relax.

Makes: 8 ounces

Ingredients

¼ cup finely ground dry coffee

½ cup sugar

½ teaspoon natural vanilla extract

2 tablespoons coconut oil

2 tablespoons castor oil

Directions

1.   Mix the coffee, sugar, and vanilla in a bowl.

2.   Gradually add the oils while mixing.

3.   Apply to problem areas and rub in a circular motion. Rinse with warm water.

Chapter 3. Cream Recipes

Anti-Wrinkle Face Cream

The rosehip seed oil in this concoction will work its regenerative and moisturizing powers on your face! Rosehip seed oil is said to enhance elastin and collagen production in the skin, helping erase fine lines and wrinkles.

Makes: 1.5 ounces. Preparation time: 45 minutes

Ingredients

2 teaspoons jojoba oil
1 teaspoon coconut oil
3 teaspoons apricot kernel oil
3 teaspoons rosehip seed oil
1 ½ teaspoons beeswax pastilles
6-10 teaspoons rose-water

Directions

1.   Place all the ingredients EXCEPT the rose water in a double boiler.

2.   Heat until melted (about 5 minutes).

3.   Remove the bowl from the heat and let it cool until it is comfortable to handle, but not solidified.

4.   Carefully transfer the mixture to a blender, and pulse while adding the rose water gradually.

5.   You should get a light, creamy mixture. Store it in a clean airtight container, in a cool place.

Anti-Acne Cream with Grapeseed Oil

Grapeseed oil is known to tighten pores and reduce oiliness while protecting the skin's natural oil barrier. Cedarwood essential oil lends its anti-inflammatory and antiseptic properties. The other ingredients, like witch hazel, vitamin E, aloe vera, and grapefruit seed extract all add to the acne-fighting and skin-conditioning qualities of this cream. Stearic acid can be of animal or plant origin, and adds to texture without adding to greasiness.

Makes: 4 ounces Preparation time: 10 minutes plus cooling time

Ingredients

4 teaspoons grapeseed oil

1 tablespoon emulsifying wax

½ teaspoon stearic acid

½ teaspoon vitamin E oil

⅓ cup witch hazel (liquid)

1 tablespoon aloe vera gel

5 drops grapefruit seed extract

5 drops lemon or lavender essential oil

1 drop cedarwood essential oil

Directions

1.   Sterilize dark, glass jars.

2.   Combine the grapeseed oil, emulsifying wax, and stearic acid in a heatproof bowl or double boiler.

3.   Heat gently over boiling water until the wax has melted.

4.   Remove the mixture from the heat and add the vitamin E oil. Stir, and set it aside.

5.   To prevent separation in the mixture, the witch hazel must not be cold when added to the oil mixture. To warm it, combine it with the aloe vera gel in a heatproof container, place it over the double boiler, and heat to lukewarm.

6.   Whisk the warmed witch hazel mixture while gradually pouring in the oil mixture in a thin stream.

7.   Continue whisking while adding the grape seed extract and the essential oils.

8.   Pour the mixture into the sterilized, dark jars and let it cool. Stir occasionally to prevent separation.

9.   Place the lids on when the mixture is completely cooled, and store it away from heat and light.

10.   Apply on the face as a night cream after cleansing.

Anti-Aging Face Cream with Rose Water, Wheat Germ & Honey

Shea butter restores the skin's moisture, while rose water rejuvenates the skin. Honey and beeswax will retain the moisture, and also help fight signs of aging. Wheat germ tightens skin cells and improves elasticity.

Makes: 7-8 ounces
Preparation time:

Ingredients

8 teaspoons beeswax, grated

4 tablespoons rose water

4 teaspoons organic honey

¼ cup shea butter

8 teaspoons wheat germ oil

4 tablespoons sweet almond oil

10 drops carrot seed oil

10 drops rose oil, or any essential oil of your choice

Directions

1.   Sterilize your containers.

2.   Place the beeswax in a glass container. Place the container in a double boiler on low heat.

3.   Pour the rose water into a separate cup, and place the cup in the double boiler, along with the beeswax. Similarly, warm the honey it its own container.

4.   When the beeswax is melted, add the shea butter and stir constantly until it melts and is well blended. Add the wheat germ oil and sweet almond oil. Whip it with a whisk or an immersion blender until everything is thoroughly combined.

5.   Keep mixing, while you add the warm rose water and warm honey, and continue to stir while the mixture cools down.

6.   Add the carrot seed oil and rose oil, and stir to combine.

7.   Transfer the mixture to your clean containers, and label them.

Soothing and Moisturizing Cream

This cream is packed with moisturizing and nourishing ingredients. Coconut oil moisturizes without suffocating the skin, while also protecting against bacteria and viruses. Tea tree oil is mildly antiseptic and effective against acne. Vetiver, though not very well known, has amazing anti-aging properties and a very pleasant aroma.

Makes: 7 ounces

Ingredients

⅓ cup shea butter
⅓ cup virgin coconut oil
¼ cup almond oil
5-7 drops vetiver essential oil
10-15 drops tea tree oil

Directions

1.   Soften the shea butter in a double boiler, or in a heatproof cup over a pot of hot water.

2.   Once softened, add the rest of the ingredients and mix thoroughly.

3.   Cover and refrigerate until the mixture has solidified.

4.   Whip with a hand mixer until a fluffy cream is formed.

5.   Pour into prepared jars. Keep it refrigerated while unused.

6.   Rub a small amount in damp hands and gently apply to the face in a circular motion.

7.   Rinse off, pat dry, and follow with a gentle moisturizer.

Moisturizer and Makeup Remover

Here's a moisturizer that's simple to make and chemical-free. It protects skin from dryness and also acts as a makeup remover.

Makes: 18 ounces

Ingredients

¾ ounce (by weight) beeswax pastilles, unscented, cosmetic grade
¼ cup sunflower oil

¼ cup coconut oil

1 cup aloe vera gel

10 drops chamomile OR lavender essential oil

Directions

1.   Melt the beeswax, sunflower oil, and coconut oil in a double boiler or chocolate melter.

2.   Pour the heated mixture into a blender, and let it cool to just a bit warmer than room temperature. It should look like a thick oil.

3.   If the aloe vera is cold, gently warm it to lukewarm. You may do this over a double boiler or by placing it in a heatproof glass measuring cup over hot water.

4.   Stir the essential oil into the heated aloe vera gel.

5.   The wax and aloe vera mixture should both be lukewarm at this point. Adding cold aloe vera to the wax mixture will result in separation.

6.   Start blending the wax mixture, scraping the bottom to ensure thorough blending.

7.   Very gradually, pour in the aloe vera mixture while blending. The mixture will turn into a white, fluffy cream.

8.   Keep a small amount for use and store the rest in the refrigerator.

Apricot Moisture Cream for Sensitive Skin

Apricot seed oil is great for sensitive skin because it's non-irritating, but gently moisturizing and nourishing. The ingredients are either non-comedogenic or have a low comedogenic rating, and are therefore perfect for sensitive skin!

Makes: 3 ounces

Ingredients

3 tablespoons shea butter

3 tablespoons apricot seed oil

½ teaspoon vitamin E oil

1 teaspoon aloe vera gel

5 drops chamomile OR rose OR neroli essential oils

Directions

1.   Using a blender or mixer with a wire whip attachment, whip the shea butter to a fluffy consistency.

2.   Gradually add the other ingredients while whipping.

3.   Transfer the mixture to a clean jar, cover tightly, and label.

Anti-Puffiness Face Cream

This cream will remove the puffiness and dark circles under your eyes. The caffeine in green tea constricts blood vessels to reduce swelling, and it also soothes inflammation and irritation. Almond oil reduces puffiness and discoloration. It will also nourish your skin and help soften or erase wrinkles. Then there's the cell-regenerative property of rosehip seed oil, and the potent moisturizing and soothing effect of carrot seed oil. It's chock-full of benefits!

Makes: 4 ounces

Ingredients

1 teaspoon emulsifying wax

1 tablespoon rosehip seed oil

¼ teaspoon vitamin E oil

1 tablespoon sweet almond oil

¼ cup brewed green tea

1 drop carrot seed essential oil

3 drops choice of essential oil (chamomile, lavender or rose)

Directions

1. Sterilize all equipment that will come in contact with the ingredients by wiping it down with rubbing alcohol and leaving it to dry completely before use.

2. Prepare two glass bowls and two medium-sized pans.

3.   Fill the pans halfway with water and place them over the stovetop.

4.   To one bowl, add the wax, rosehip seed oil, vitamin E oil, and sweet almond oil.

5.   Pour the brewed green tea into the other bowl.

6.   Place one bowl over each water-filled pan and turn on to medium heat.

7.   Heat to 130°F. The content of both bowls should be the same temperature, or else the cream will not set.

8.   Pour the green tea into the wax mixture.

9.   Whip the mixture with a handheld mixer or blender.

10.   Blending should be intermittent and can take 30 minutes to an hour before the water is no longer separated from the oils.

11.   When it reaches a light, creamy consistency, stir in the carrot seed and other essential oils.

12.   Pour into sterilized containers.

Bonus Chapter. Autumn Essential Blends.

There are a list of essential oils you can use for your skin to help it look younger and healthier.

Cautions and Care

An essential oil is the most potent form of any plant; however, there are a few things you need to know about essential oils before you begin to use them.

1. Can cause contact dermatitis when used un-diluted. There are websites out there that will tell it is alright not to dilute the oils. This is false.

2. If you are not sure whether your skin will have a reaction to the use of certain essential oils, you can go to your nearest store that sells them and ask for a patch test. This will help you determine which essential oils will be alright for you to use.

3. Store the essential oils in a cool, dry place. Many essential oils are very light and will evaporate when exposed to heat.

4. Store your scrubs in tightly lidded dark glass containers to prevent light from entering and possibly heating up the mixture.

5. Scrubs have the same shelf life as the sugar you used to make them. It is best not to keep them longer than that. For maximum potency, use them after letting sit overnight in the container.

6. Do not apply scrubs to cracked, raw skin or open wounds. It will irritate the area to which it is applied.

The list

Bergamot, Citrus bergamia This one is good for treating cold sores as well as acne, and greasy skin.

Cedarwood, Texas, Juniperus ashei This is the first of two types of Cedarwood that are used for skin issues. This help with oily skin, it also helps with acne, eczema, psoriasis.

Cedarwood, Virginian, Juniperus virginiana This essential oil is also good for the same things of its relative. The difference is, being a different genus, it can be gentler than the Texas version.

Chamomile, Roman, Chamaemelum nobile This is an especially good essential oil for acne, eczema, light rashes, dermatitis, and inflammations.

Clary Sage, salvia sclarea This is an essential oil that is good for regulating oily skin, and also helping to reduce swelling and fight acne. It's good for wrinkles, too.

Clove Bud, Syzygium armaticum This is good for stubborn acne.

Galbanum, Ferula galbaniflua This helps to heal scar tissue, tones skin, wrinkles as well as acne.

Geranium, Pelargonium graveolens This essential oil is excellent for speeding the healing of broken capillaries, acne, burns, helps to unclog pores, and balances an oily complexion.

Grapefruit, Citrus x paradisi This essential oil helps to tone and reduce sagging in skin and skin. It helps to unclog pore and regulate skin. It is also good for acne.

Helichrysum, Helichrysum angutifolium This essential oil can help with inflammations of the skin caused by rosacea and puffiness around the eyes, chin and other problem areas. It has also been used to help treat acne, dermatitis, eczema, and age spots and blemishes for pinched zits.

Juniper, Juniperus communis

This essential oil is used to help treat acne breakouts and existing pimples. It has also been used to help treat skin conditions such as dermatitis and rosacea. It is also a skin toner.

Lavender, Lavendula angustifolia

This is an all-around essential oil for promoting healthy skin. It helps to reduce blemishes and scarring and helps to speed healing of acne that has been pinched. It also has antiseptic properties.

Lime, Citrus aurantifolia This is another good one for spots in the skin, warts, greasy skin, and acne.

Myrtle, Myrtus communis This essential oil is highly recommended for treating oily skin and it helps to open pours for a deeper cleansing.

Naouli, Melaluca viridiflora This is another oil that is good for treating oily skin and all types of acne.

Palmarosa, Cymbopogon martinii var. martinii Another essential oil that helps to reduce scarring and wrinkles, it is also recommended for acne, dry skin conditions. It also helps to moisturize the skin.

Patchouli, Pogostemon cablin This is essential is used for a very wide array of skin conditions. Not only does it treat acne, it also helps with rosacea, dermatitis, eczema, fungal infections, oily skin, helps to shrink open pores, and wrinkles.

Peppermint, Mentha piperita This essential oil has antiseptic properties. It is also good for treating acne.

Rosemary, Rosmarinus officinalis This is one that is not recommended if you have hypertension as it can raise the blood pressure. It is used mainly for acne, dermatitis, and eczema.

Rosewood, Aniba rosaeodora This essential oil helps to bring combination complexions into balance. It is also good for general, everyday skin care. It is good for regular and sensitive skin.

Sandalwood, Santalum album Helps to regulate greasy skin and can be an efficient moisturizer. This is also good for acne.

Tea Tree, Melaluca Alternifolia Because of its aroma, it is used in small does, but it is a potent skin toner and treatment for acne. It also helps to treat oily skin.

There are more essential oils than this on the market, but these are the ones I highly recommend for scrubs.

Thyme, Thymus Vulgaris Like many others, it helps to regulate oily skin and fight acne. Thyme should be avoided when pregnant. Overuse can lead to sensitivity of the essential oil.

Vetiver, Vetiveria zizanioe This essential oil helps to combat acne and oily skin. *Violet*, Viola odorata Violet essential oil helps to refine pours, smooth out eczema, and treat acne.

Yarrow, Achillea millefolium This essential oil helps to tone the skin as well as treat skin conditions like eczema, inflammations, and rashes. It also helps to treat acne.

Ylang Ylang, Canaga odorata var. genuina This is another essential oil for general skin care. It helps with irritated and inflamed skin. Also helps treat acne, and oily skin.

Combining Essential Oils

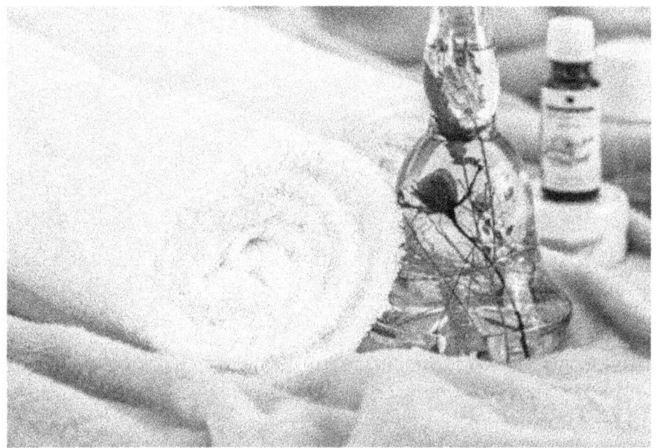

There are three types of essential oils:

Light
Medium,
And heavy.

These are usually known as "notes". When combining them, you will generally use more of the light and medium than you would the heavy. Making blends is usually in small batches, one tablespoon at a time.

Magic Musky Moonlight

8 drops cardamom
7 drops cedar
5 drops calamus

Combine all the oils together in a glass jar, or directly into your diffuser. Fill your diffuser with water according to the size of your diffuser.

You can follow the recipe here as is, or you can feel free to modify to your own personal preference. Whatever you decide to do, have fun with it and love your blend!

Spice Cake Surprise

6 drops cinnamon
6 drops clove oil
5 drops garlic oil
7 drops chamomile

Combine all the oils together in a glass jar, or directly into your diffuser. Fill your diffuser with water according to the size of your diffuser.

You can follow the recipe here as is, or you can feel free to modify to your own personal preference. Whatever you decide to do, have fun with it and love your blend!

The Dessert Spice Blend

6 drops clary sage
8 drops sandalwood
5 drops ginger

Combine all the oils together in a glass jar, or directly into your diffuser. Fill your diffuser with water according to the size of your diffuser.

You can follow the recipe here as is, or you can feel free to modify to your own personal preference. Whatever you decide to do, have fun with it and love your blend!

The Wood Fairies

5 drops rosewood
5 drops cedar wood
8 drops sandalwood
5 drops pine

Combine all the oils together in a glass jar, or directly into your diffuser. Fill your diffuser with water according to the size of your diffuser.

You can follow the recipe here as is, or you can feel free to modify to your own personal preference. Whatever you decide to do, have fun with it and love your blend!

Magic Music

6 drops jasmine
5 drops hyssop
5 drops neem oil

Combine all the oils together in a glass jar, or directly into your diffuser. Fill your diffuser with water according to the size of your diffuser.

You can follow the recipe here as is, or you can feel free to modify to your own personal preference. Whatever you decide to do, have fun with it and love your blend!

The Richness of the Earth

7 drops patchouli
5 drops red cedar
4 drops lemongrass
2 drops rosehip

Combine all the oils together in a glass jar, or directly into your diffuser. Fill your diffuser with water according to the size of your diffuser.

You can follow the recipe here as is, or you can feel free to modify to your own personal preference. Whatever you decide to do, have fun with it and love your blend!

A Walk Around The Block

4 drops cedar

4 drops cedarwood

5 drops clary sage

5 drops sage

Combine all the oils together in a glass jar, or directly into your diffuser. Fill your diffuser with water according to the size of your diffuser.

You can follow the recipe here as is, or you can feel free to modify to your own personal preference. Whatever you decide to do, have fun with it and love your blend!

Bees and Butterflies

6 drops spruce

6 drops tangerine

6 drops pine

Combine all the oils together in a glass jar, or directly into your diffuser. Fill your diffuser with water according to the size of your diffuser.

You can follow the recipe here as is, or you can feel free to modify to your own personal preference. Whatever you decide to do, have fun with it and love your blend!

The Gently Blowing Breeze

8 drops patchouli
8 drops lemongrass
4 drops tea tree
5 drops tarragon

Combine all the oils together in a glass jar, or directly into your diffuser. Fill your diffuser with water according to the size of your diffuser.

You can follow the recipe here as is, or you can feel free to modify to your own personal preference. Whatever you decide to do, have fun with it and love your blend!

Fresh Linen on the Line

5 drops peppermint
5 drops eucalyptus
6 drops tangerine
5 drops spearmint

Combine all the oils together in a glass jar, or directly into your diffuser. Fill your diffuser with water according to the size of your diffuser.

You can follow the recipe here as is, or you can feel free to modify to your own personal preference. Whatever you decide to do, have fun with it and love your blend!

Raindrops on the Roses

10 drops eucalyptus
8 drops rosewood
8 drops rose
5 drops sage

Combine all the oils together in a glass jar, or directly into your diffuser. Fill your diffuser with water according to the size of your diffuser.

You can follow the recipe here as is, or you can feel free to modify to your own personal preference. Whatever you decide to do, have fun with it and love your blend!

The Flower Garden

10 drops lavender
10 drops rose
6 drops hibiscus
6 drops lilac
5 drops lemon
5 drops tangerine

Combine all the oils together in a glass jar, or directly into your diffuser. Fill your diffuser with water according to the size of your diffuser.

You can follow the recipe here as is, or you can feel free to modify to your own personal preference. Whatever you decide to do, have fun with it and love your blend!

Umbrella on my Shoulders

10 drops orange
5 drops blood orange
5 drops lime oil
4 drops eucalyptus

Combine all the oils together in a glass jar, or directly into your diffuser. Fill your diffuser with water according to the size of your diffuser.

You can follow the recipe here as is, or you can feel free to modify to your own personal preference. Whatever you decide to do, have fun with it and love your blend!

The Headache Buster

10 drops peppermint
10 drops eucalyptus
5 drops wintergreen
5 drops spearmint

Combine all the oils together in a glass jar, or directly into your diffuser. Fill your diffuser with water according to the size of your diffuser.

You can follow the recipe here as is, or you can feel free to modify to your own personal preference. Whatever you decide to do, have fun with it and love your blend!

The Immunity Booster

5 drops frankincense
4 drops lemon
4 drops eucalyptus
5 drops garlic
10 drops tea tree

Combine all the oils together in a glass jar, or directly into your diffuser. Fill your diffuser with water according to the size of your diffuser.

You can follow the recipe here as is, or you can feel free to modify to your own personal preference. Whatever you decide to do, have fun with it and love your blend!

The Calming Blend

10 drops vetiver
5 drops lavender
5 drops peppermint
2 drops spearmint

Combine all the oils together in a glass jar, or directly into your diffuser. Fill your diffuser with water according to the size of your diffuser.

You can follow the recipe here as is, or you can feel free to modify to your own personal preference. Whatever you decide to do, have fun with it and love your blend!

The Life of the Party

10 drops lemongrass
4 drops lemon
4 drops tangerine
5 drops sweet orange
5 drops orange

Combine all the oils together in a glass jar, or directly into your diffuser. Fill your diffuser with water according to the size of your diffuser.

You can follow the recipe here as is, or you can feel free to modify to your own personal preference. Whatever you decide to do, have fun with it and love your blend!

The Fixer Fizzer

8 drops tea tree
8 drops peppermint
4 drops myrrh
4 drops cardamom

Combine all the oils together in a glass jar, or directly into your diffuser. Fill your diffuser with water according to the size of your diffuser.

You can follow the recipe here as is, or you can feel free to modify to your own personal preference. Whatever you decide to do, have fun with it and love your blend!

The All In One Blend

5 drops goldenseal
10 drops grapefruit
4 drops ginger
4 drops cinnamon

Combine all the oils together in a glass jar, or directly into your diffuser. Fill your diffuser with water according to the size of your diffuser.

You can follow the recipe here as is, or you can feel free to modify to your own personal preference. Whatever you decide to do, have fun with it and love your blend!

Aches and Pains Melt Away Blend

11 drops lavender
11 drops spruce
5 drops cedar wood
5 drops grapefruit

Combine all the oils together in a glass jar, or directly into your diffuser. Fill your diffuser with water according to the size of your diffuser.

You can follow the recipe here as is, or you can feel free to modify to your own personal preference. Whatever you decide to do, have fun with it and love your blend!

The Bedroom Blend

10 drops peppermint
5 drops cinnamon
5 drops wintergreen
5 drops spruce

Combine all the oils together in a glass jar, or directly into your diffuser. Fill your diffuser with water according to the size of your diffuser.

You can follow the recipe here as is, or you can feel free to modify to your own personal preference. Whatever you decide to do, have fun with it and love your blend!

Yours Truly Blend

10 drops rose
8 drops lavender
3 drops spearmint
3 drops grapefruit
3 drops tea tree oil

Combine all the oils together in a glass jar, or directly into your diffuser. Fill your diffuser with water according to the size of your diffuser.

You can follow the recipe here as is, or you can feel free to modify to your own personal preference. Whatever you decide to do, have fun with it and love your blend!

Anything and Everything

8 drops frankincense
4 drops spikenard
4 drops patchouli
4 drops vetiver
3 drops spruce

Combine all the oils together in a glass jar, or directly into your diffuser. Fill your diffuser with water according to the size of your diffuser.

You can follow the recipe here as is, or you can feel free to modify to your own personal preference. Whatever you decide to do, have fun with it and love your blend!

Everything You Wanted Blend

9 drops ylang ylang
5 drops tangerine
5 drops wintergreen
4 drops cedar wood

Combine all the oils together in a glass jar, or directly into your diffuser. Fill your diffuser with water according to the size of your diffuser.

You can follow the recipe here as is, or you can feel free to modify to your own personal preference. Whatever you decide to do, have fun with it and love your blend!

You and Me is Three Blend

4 drops tea tree
8 drops grapefruit
8 drops cinnamon

Combine all the oils together in a glass jar, or directly into your diffuser. Fill your diffuser with water according to the size of your diffuser.

You can follow the recipe here as is, or you can feel free to modify to your own personal preference. Whatever you decide to do, have fun with it and love your blend!

Your Dream Come True Blend

8 drops lavender
9 drops spruce
4 drops ylang ylang
3 drops tea tree

Combine all the oils together in a glass jar, or directly into your diffuser. Fill your diffuser with water according to the size of your diffuser.

You can follow the recipe here as is, or you can feel free to modify to your own personal preference. Whatever you decide to do, have fun with it and love your blend!

The Super Spoiler Blend

12 drops ylang ylang
6 drops vetiver
4 drops myrrh
4 drops patchouli

Combine all the oils together in a glass jar, or directly into your diffuser. Fill your diffuser with water according to the size of your diffuser.

You can follow the recipe here as is, or you can feel free to modify to your own personal preference. Whatever you decide to do, have fun with it and love your blend!

Indulgence in Love Blend

7 drops cinnamon
4 drops rose
4 drops tangerine
2 drops spearmint
2 drops tea tree oil

Combine all the oils together in a glass jar, or directly into your diffuser. Fill your diffuser with water according to the size of your diffuser.

You can follow the recipe here as is, or you can feel free to modify to your own personal preference. Whatever you decide to do, have fun with it and love your blend!

Good Day Blend

5 drops rosewood
3 drops lemon
3 drops lemongrass

Combine all the oils together in a glass jar, or directly into your diffuser. Fill your diffuser with water according to the size of your diffuser.

You can follow the recipe here as is, or you can feel free to modify to your own personal preference. Whatever you decide to do, have fun with it and love your blend!

The Candyshop Blend

5 drops peppermint
3 drops lemon
3 drops rose
1 drop lavender

Combine all the oils together in a glass jar, or directly into your diffuser. Fill your diffuser with water according to the size of your diffuser.

You can follow the recipe here as is, or you can feel free to modify to your own personal preference. Whatever you decide to do, have fun with it and love your blend!

Money for my Honey

6 drops goldenseal
5 drops frankincense
3 drops rosewood

Combine all the oils together in a glass jar, or directly into your diffuser. Fill your diffuser with water according to the size of your diffuser.

You can follow the recipe here as is, or you can feel free to modify to your own personal preference. Whatever you decide to do, have fun with it and love your blend!

Fluffy Clouds

8 drops myrrh
5 drops goldenseal
3 drops orange

Combine all the oils together in a glass jar, or directly into your diffuser. Fill your diffuser with water according to the size of your diffuser.

You can follow the recipe here as is, or you can feel free to modify to your own personal preference. Whatever you decide to do, have fun with it and love your blend!

Peaceful Blend

8 drops agar
5 drops anise
5 drops rose

Combine all the oils together in a glass jar, or directly into your diffuser. Fill your diffuser with water according to the size of your diffuser.

Conclusion

Take the first attempts as a learning experience but figure out the adjustments and changes you need to make for your next batch of soap. Don't be scared of sharing your experiences with others, and if you know someone who is good at making soap, ask them for suggestions. Anyone and everyone can make soap. It just requires some practice. And when you become a professional, help out the beginners by telling them your experiences and sharing your ups and downs.

Since we have learned how to make soaps, creams and Scrubs, I hope that you will apply the acquired knowledge productively. Thank you.